LOGISTICS OF LEANNESS DEFINED

LOGISTICS OF LEANNESS DEFINED

By Leigh Hickombottom

Pictures taken by Mike Anthony Moffa.
Book Cover Design: Lulu.com Professional Services
Designer: Kent Swecker, A New Machine

ISBN 978-0-557-25442-2

Visit www.Logisticsofleanness.com
and www.Holleighwood.com

*This booklet is dedicated to my daughters Kierra and Tatjana.
Live your dreams my sweethearts. You can be anything
your heart desires. Believe! ;0)*

CONTENTS

THE OPENING

FITNESS = LIFESTYLE My equation, my reality for successful weight management

365 day a year lifestyle. Continued success without the rollercoaster weight loss game of yo-yo dieting is derived from this formula. That is what it is all about and that is what it takes to be successful with this weight loss program. My personal success stems from making my health and fitness apart of my everyday routine. Getting to this physique began with having a goal. Maintaining this physique moves beyond reaching the goal once accomplished. A sustain physique calls for a whole new way of living, a lifestyle.

In Logistics of Leanness you were given a general look into my secrets and my personal cardio regimen. This time around I will define the importance of your mind along with actual resistance training for the overall tone of the body. Also given are a few reminders from the first booklet. Alright, SUPERWOMEN and SUPERMEN now that you are ready to ROCK let's get started!

The base… The foundation… is your mind. This is the core, the essence of what this lifestyle is about for me. You have heard that mind over matter and mind and body connection saying. The fore front of this weight management success begins and ends with the mind. Yes, it is that important. Visualize, Visualize, Visualize. Your mind will get your body to where you desire it to be. This with good positive loving feelings not only amplifies your results, it delivers lasting results. Believe in yourself. Know that you will and can obtain any body image you wish with positive thinking and visualization.

POWER OF THE MIND

There is what some of you may have already heard or read about called the LAW of ATTRACTION. For me, this exists whether you believe in it or not. This is a given. It is kind of like gravity to me. Whether or not I can actually see the pull of gravity or not (which I am not able to see) it exists. While I will not go into grave detail for this book I will share in short, what is needed for you to better understand the purpose behind this "LAW". Understanding this "LAW" will help you to fully understand the importance of your mind, your thoughts and actions.

You will understand the UNIVERSAL LAW/ LAW of ATTRACTION and why it is so important to me and my fitness regimen. This will also let you in on why this needs to be a fundamental element in achieving your goal.

The short of UNIVERSAL LAW….. Our thoughts, our feelings, our words and our actions are a form of energy, thus, creating our reality. So why not use this to our advantage and create our ideal body image. Restructure your mind to be open to this. You think positive and the result is that SUPERWOMAN and SUPERMAN like physique. Negative thoughts set you up for an automatic failure, meaning dissatisfied results. Since we are SUPERWOMEN and SUPERMEN failure is not an option :0)

What you focus your mind upon you attract. The universe manifests the positive thoughts as well as the not so positive. This is why it is important to focus on the ideal image of our new bodies as opposed to the current dissatisfied one. If I am always focused (complaining) about that jiggle in my thighs or how big they appear I am putting ENERGY on this flaw. Not realizing the universe has no idea that I do not like this flaw. The universe does know I am giving this area of my body ENERGY (attention) as is and therefore thinks I wish to keep it as it is. Why else would I be putting ENERGY on this?? The result of this thought process equals the body remaining the same if not appearing worse due to focusing too much ENERGY on the flaw.

Your mind is a great tool once you understand this. Focus your mind and visualizations not on your current flaws when you look in the mirror. Instead focus on that perfect body image you desire to attain as if it is you at this moment. Feel, believe and know this is you right now.

This may be hard in the beginning but it gets easier with time and with repetition. SUPERWOMEN and SUPERMEN must focus our minds on the positive thoughts only. In doing so, positive results are attained. Got it?? GOOD! :0) Go into your lifestyle change knowing, I mean really knowing, you have already succeeded. Doubt free the universe delivers to you on a GOLDEN platter... Your Ideal Image in the flesh :0)

Yes, you still have to put in the physical work during this process; however this is the easy part. Believe me when I say the physical work is 10 times easier than trying to gain full control of your mind. You controlling your mind will be the actual hard part. This is not as easy as it sounds. But hey, Now you have a heads up :0)

Just as an example I will prove it to you. Stop reading for a moment, sit still and try to get your mind still....No thoughts whatsoever for a couple of minutes! Go ahead I'll wait...

Welcome back. Not so easy is it?? For how long was your mind totally clear with no thoughts at all??? Extremely short, I know. Our minds are very busy and we must learn to gain control of it.

It is quite easy to have thoughts other than positive ones pop up in our heads. Start ignoring them. See yourself healthy and toned wearing that 2-piecefor women and swim trunks without a shirt for the men. Picture yourself looking HOTT!! You can do it SUPERWOMEN and SUPERMEN!! At this point, we are going to move into the Leigh gym mentality.

THE SWITCH FROM MY POINT TODAY

When I am at the gym, my demeanor when walking through that door, in between my sets and even upon my exit from the gym is completely different from when I am actually exercising. My mind is 100% focused while performing my exercises and in the moment of each set.

Those of you have spent at least 10mins in my presence know that I am playful about 95% of the time. So usually you will find me smiling and laughing. This includes in between sets as well. This part of my everyday personality makes it part of my lifestyle. Thus leading me to the "SWITCH" which I will come back to in a few minutes and give you more detail about.

When I say that my demeanor is different at certain times throughout my gym visit it is because of the way I start before I actually perform the exercises. The following is my start before even picking up a weight and executing.

Before I start any resistance exercise I drop my head for a moment, briefly close my eyes, take three deep breaths then visualize. My quick but important visualization is of me perfectly performing my reputations for the set I am getting ready to perform. I see myself performing to my fullest capability in proper form and fulfilling my personal repetition goal.

I then open my eyes and execute as if there was not one person in the gym other than myself for that given moment. A visual of what I see is this.... In that moment of executing the exercise, there is only movement of my body and the end result of what that portion of the body in which I am exercising looks like at the end of that repetition. The end result of what that body part should look like is my goal or ideal image as a result of performing these exercises.

This requires a different frame of mind for me. Starting from this moment I am focused, I am strong and every thought and action performed right before and during exercise is performed in pure PERFECTION. This for me requires my mind moving away from the playfulness and friendliness to an I mean business and I am unstoppable frame of mind.

Thus bring us back to the "SWTICH" I mentioned earlier. This is it for me. It is my frame of mind turned on to focus mode. I am in complete body and mind ONENESS. The focus switch I can turn on and off in a matter of seconds. Like most people I too have a very busy mind. In the beginning the switch was not so easy for me to operate. Understand everyone is different and while now after years of practice this switch is easy to control; it was not always as easy to control. Let's just say I had to turn the SWITCH on before I even walked into the gym. I actually started turning the SWITCH on right after I put my exercise gear on.

For some of you this switch that I easily turn on/off in a matter of seconds today, may actually be accomplished on your first try. For others like myself, it takes getting used to. Practice! Practice! Practice!

Yes, Practice does make perfect.

Before I give you where I personally started, I would like for you to attempt to start from where I am currently. Our minds are extremely powerful. You at this point have more information about the mind and UNIVERSAL LAW then I was given at the time. I had to learn and experience for myself to gain this understanding.

For a few days start from where I am at this point in my life with the switch. I have 100% confidence that if you believe as strongly as I do in your ability to start from this point and run with it, you will be successful from this point. Clear your mind, breathe and believe in yourself. Your thought process as I continually state is vital!! You have either already succeeded before you have begun or not. The success ALL, I mean ALL begins and ends with you! So jump to it! :0)

Now for those of you who have attempted and feel you need a gradual build into that step that is fine as well. There are no real failures here with this. Your success and timing of you reaching your success is determined by where you are at this point of your life with your control over your mind. So let's put on a big Leigh Texas sized smile on and get started with my beginning.

THE SWITCH FROM MY BEGINNINGS

In the beginning, I started with a super busy mind frame. I mean my mind was in overdrive all day until bedtime. I had to start focusing early for my gym workouts. This for me was 30-45 minutes before I actually walked into the gym. Yes, this was a long 30- 45 minutes of time to prepare to focus on the workout I would have once I walked into the gym. At least I thought so at the time. Preparing myself to prepare once at my destination was hard work for me.

Here is the visual for you... Leigh is all suited up for the gym and now turns her SWITCH on to focused mode. The funny thing about this SWITCH during this time is that there were what appeared to be glitches at first. I would turn on my SWITCH fully and the SWITCH would decide to only partially turn on as to override me fully turning it on. So while I would turn this SWITCH on to level 10, The SWITCH would magically move only to level 5 or 7. Funny thing, that switch. I literally for a while would be in a mode to half or somewhat focused before the gym. Having to train my mind daily that I was the boss! Did I say this process took me a while? :0)

During this time my normal bubbly and playful personality was set aside. The serious SUPERWOMAN side of me was called into action. This focused side of me has the goal positioned directly in front of me in full, attainable view. Any road blocks on the path to this goal are single handedly thrown aside by the tougher, serious, and determined Leigh.

This entails Leigh going to the gym with the determination to get my mind and muscle as one. I am focused about my workout coming up in the next 30-45 mins and the outcome of my body as a result of this best workout ever. I go into the gym knowing that every workout each and every time I walk into the gym is the best workout I have ever had. The reason is as a result of this workout I am both stronger and toner.

Focused on these great results and my ideal body image for 30 mins, I head to the gym. For you SUPERWOMEN, I have my "sale" shopping face on. For the SUPERMEN, my football game face is on!

That was my start leading to the gym with the SWITCH. Opposed to my quick turn on power now, I had to prepare to prepare. This was done as early as 45minutes before walking into the gym. You are not alone. You gradually build from where you feel comfortable. Do not be hard on yourself. Controlling the mind takes the majority of people time to conquer. All it takes is PRACTICE :0)

Side note Once you have accomplished turning your switch on/off you will be able to use this in every aspect of your life. This use right now is for weight management. You now have an additional plus to getting the switch method down. :0)

AFFIRMATIONS

* Affirmation: To declare as true Saying affirmations keeps your mind focused and lets the universe know this is your desire. By you focusing your mind on your ideal image, you are giving this image (the new you) energy. This is what we want to do. Incorporating affirmations with visualizations makes your visualizations more powerful. Remember you are changing your old frame of thinking. You are now refocusing your energy away from this dissatisfied image to the new jaw dropping image you actually desire.

Affirmations work extremely well for me. I have an affirmation I use during my weight loss period and still today to maintain. This affirmation is said a minimum of 10 times a day silently or out loud. This will be an added bonus to help get you where you desire to be. Try adding this to the plan. This is the affirmation I used. Feel free to use it as is or change it to make it more personal.

I am a healthy, happy _____lbs of perfect leanness. (My image of perfect leanness might be different from yours. Picture that image, that perfect image of you in your visualization)

This is short, positive and to the point. You fill in the blank space with your ideal weight.

CHANGE THE EATING

Okay, from the day you choose to start a regimen you must also choose to change your eating habits. What you have been putting in your mouth all this time is what got you where you are today. Let's change that. This is an all or nothing move. There is no working your way to eating good; its cold turkey! By cold turkey I mean 5 days a week of healthy clean eating. On the other 2 days you are allowed to have one cheat meal. ONE! Do NOT make this an all day reward. I recommend this reward meal once in the middle of the week and the other reward at the end of the week. This Cheat meal is just as important as the structured meals the other 5 days of the week.

Now say goodbye to the unhealthy foods and overindulgences. It is time to replace these pastimes with healthier and lighter foods eaten in moderation. Those SUPER HUMAN bodies deserve the best fuel (food) available. Time to get in gear for training.

LEIGH'S SETS FOR EACH EXERCISE

I perform 2 sets for each exercise with 1 minute breaks. By doing this I get in and out of the gym and get a feeling that I have worked twice as hard as the person who has done 3 sets. Use the 2 sets for 3 weeks then we need to incorporate change. You will change both the intensity and speed after 3 weeks. Your body will continually show improvements because it is kept guessing. Plateauing will be next to impossible during this time.

With the mind fully focused stay in the moment of the training. Your 1st set needs to be at a resistance where you can perform 15-20 controlled repetitions without too much ease. By the time you have hit your last 5 repetitions you need to feel as though your muscles are fully engaged. Training the muscles hard enough to feel tension but not enough to strain or hurt yourself.

If you have ever carried out exercises consisting of 3 sets repetitions the feeling you obtain is exactly the same. During the 1st set you should feel as though you are performing a 2nd set out of a 3 set exercise. This means you need to be just as focused and controlled with the movements as if you already performed a 1st set out of a 3 set exercise. This would have you at a point of working harder than your normal 1st set.

The 2nd set has you working as if you are on your 3rd set of a normal 3 set exercise. Your muscles should be fatigued and your body working 3times as hard. Still execution needs to be controlled and you must perform 15 repetitions minimal and 20 maximum. Your resistance needs to be adjusted accordingly.

CHANGES TO INCORPORATE EVERY 2-3 WEEKS WITH YOUR SETS

These are just a few of the ways I actually change in my every day workouts to keep my body guessing.

Please note there are 30 second breaks between set 1 and 2. After performing these changes you will see/feel why it is not necessary to perform 3 sets all the time.

Change 1:

1st Set: Use weight that you can rep 15-20 times. When you hit your 15-20 rep mark, drop the weight by one weight. Perform this for another 12 reps.

2nd set: use the weight you started with in your first set and rep this for 15. Drop a weight and rep this for 10 reps. After the 10 reps drop one more weight and rep it out until you feel the burn.

Change 2:

1st Set: Use weight that you can rep a max of 10 with real effort and rep this amount for 10 reps. without pause, move up a weight and rep this 5-8 times.

2nd Set: Use the weight you used to rep 5-8 times in the first set and rep this amount for 10 reps. then drop one weight quickly and rep for 10 more.

Change 3:

1et Set: Use a weight you can only rep 10-12 times and rep this amount 10-12 times. Quickly drop by 2 weights and perform the exercise on a three count both ways (both the resistance and negative). You will rep this 10 times. This means it should take you a total of 6 seconds to complete one rep once you have dropped your weights by 2.

2nd Set: We are going to do the same as above. This will just be performed in the opposite order.

The last weight you used will be used again for another 3 count both ways for 10 reps. then quickly jump back up by two weights (this should be what you began with in the first set) and perform another 10 reps.

*Only 2 sets performed for each exercise
SUPERHEROS!! Make them count!*

YOU CHOOSE YOUR SPEED

Performing these two set require your mind to be fully focused and in the moment of the movement. This is the reason you choose your speed and intensity. For 3 weeks you will choose either the slow movement or fast movement. The following 3 weeks you will uses the movement you did not choose for the first 3 weeks.

Slow- controlled movement 4 - 5 seconds from beginning to the end of repetition.

Fast- controlled faster movement for a count of 2 - 3 seconds.

Interchange every 2 - 3 weeks as to keep our bodies in a constant mode of producing great results.

You set the tempo, your own! Your body follows. Each exercise whether slow or fast must be a controlled movement.

On that 3rd week if not done by the 2nd week you are required to change the speed of movement.

Before the change you will get stronger each week. In saying this, make sure you are feeling the exercises in your second week. You do not want these exercises to feel super easy so make sure to adjust your resistance during the 2nd week by moving up one in weight. Not done to bulk you up but to keep the body dishing out results.

At the 3rd week mark, if you started with a slow range of motion you will now change this to a fast range of motion. This means if you were performing a 4 count you will now perform at a 2-3 count. The same follows for those of you who started at a fast range of motion. You will now change the count by adding 1 - 2 seconds. Controlled and fluid range of motion remains the one constant.

You will notice the difference each of the weeks you change your tempo. The change will be both your tone and strength. I am amazed to see my body each time I have changed the tempo. The feeling I get is of my body performing each exercise for the first time even if I was at the speed a couple of weeks ago. This lets me know something very reassuring. My body is not used to performing these exercises. As a result the results I Love! Love! Love!

BEFORE THE RESISTANCE EXERCISES

Alright, on the road to the actual physical work :0) I will give you a few of my resistance exercises taken from my daily workouts. All of these exercises can be adjusted to your environment and your capabilities. Likewise, with the cardio regimen as given in Logistics of Leanness, the resistance also entails interchanging of these exercises which include the movements, machines and positions.

I will give you 2 exercises for each part of the body. These exercises are to be changed in some form or fashion every 3 weeks SUPERHEROS! You will notice by changing the exercises or by training the muscles differently every 3 weeks you will consistently see results. This is what we all want…results! No plateauing.

Focus during these exercises. As you perform your movements your mind needs to be focused on the muscle toning. Mind and body need to be in total oneness. BREATHE!

Leigh Visual…

Let's say I am training my legs. While I am performing walking lunges, fixed in my mind is the toned image of my legs already at the ideal image of what I desire my legs to look like.

Start off doing this for about a month. You will notice with your own eyes the transformation. Your bodies will start to look like that ideal image you are holding in your mind.

Important note on this technique BELIEVE! Whatever it is that you so desire, SUPERWOMEN and SUPERMEN, your physique to be, it will be. If you do not truly believe in the power of yourself, your mind and its abilities, then you have already set yourself up for failure. Failure meaning undesired results.

Your body is your own and 100% unique. Understand this. You can still have the image of that ideal body that you cut out of the magazine as you learned from Logistics of Leanness. But this image is really used to get you motivated and your mind focused. That person's body is also their own and unique to them. At the end of this your body will be hotter than what you ever imagined it could be. You will be pleased at this point that someone else's picture was just what it was… Their body used for your focus and motivation.

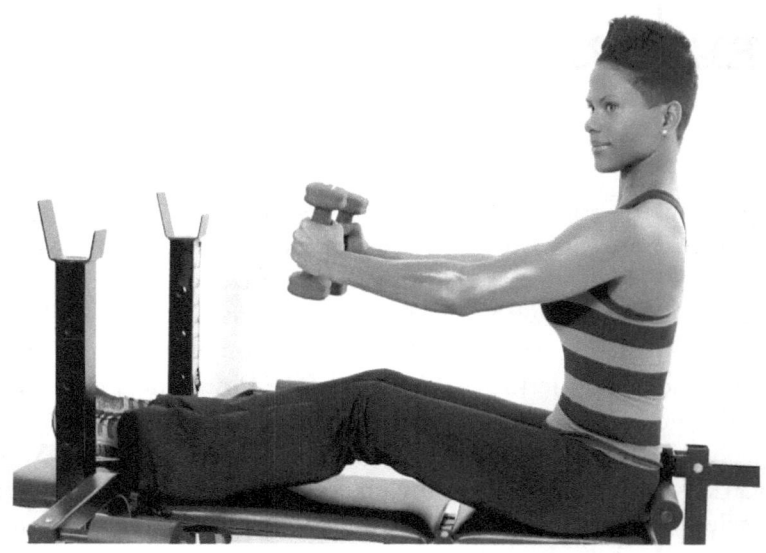

START

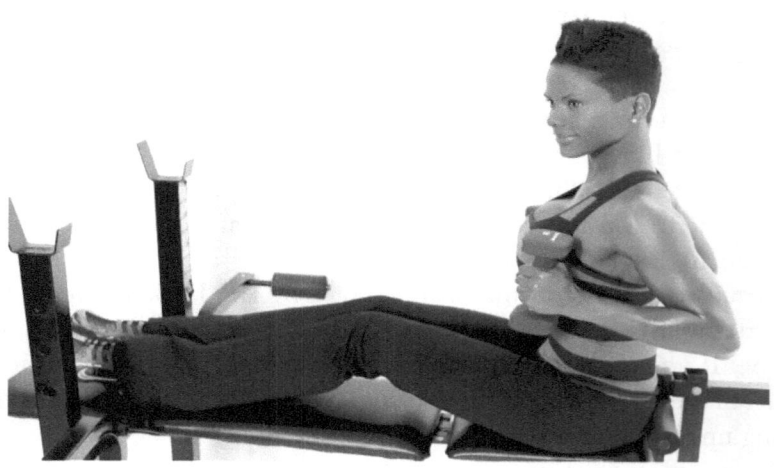

FINISH

WORKOUTS

Back

This is my favorite part of the body to train.

Seated cable rows- Great for toning the upper and middle part of the back. In the gym there are a couple of ways to perform this exercise. The first option involves and actual seated cable machine. I use the triangle handle for this. First, place the machine resistance on a weight you can perform for a controlled set of 15 repetitions. Your starting position is holding the triangle at a fully extended arms length position. Sit with the back at a fully straight position as if your back was up against a wall. Next, place your feet on the foot pedals remaining in the straight back position with the knees slightly bent. Pull the cable towards your chest while squeezing the back muscles then extend your arms back to your full arms length (start position). The completion of this first set should feel as though you have completed two full sets of repetitions.

* Your back should not arch during this exercise

* Your bottom should not jump off of the seat. If this happens your weight is too heavy. Adjust weight to a lighter resistance.

Seated row machine- The second way to perform this is at the seated row machine. There is no cable here.

Starting position has your chest up against the pad, your back is straight, and arms fully extended with hands on inner grips. You will pull the handles toward your chest, and then extend back to start position. We are using controlled movements.

For those of you without the gym memberships or who want to perform the cable row without machines, this is for you...

Seated Barbell row-Sit on the floor with legs slightly bent arms forward and back straight. Use dumbbells the resistance of your choice for this exercise. Arms need to be positioned straight in front of you. Your arms will parallel your legs which are also straight in front of you bent slightly with your feet flat on the floor.

With your arms in straight in front of you pull the dumbbells in towards the side of your chest area. Squeeze the muscles as you pull toward you then fully extend arms back to start position. Your feet and legs will be the stability needed to perform correct controlled movements.

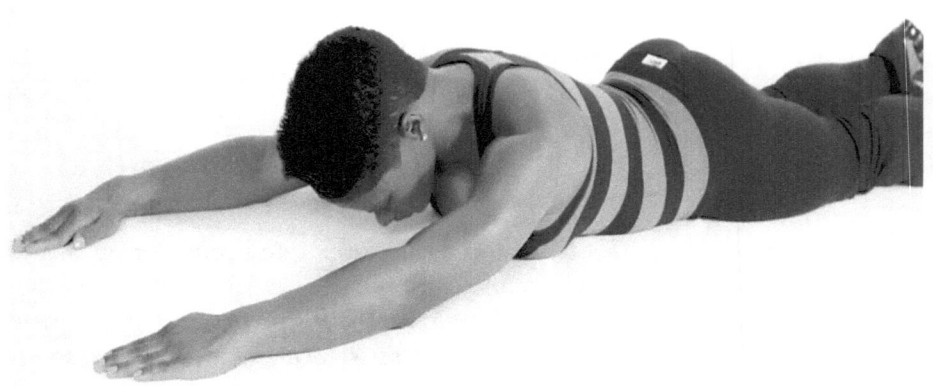

START

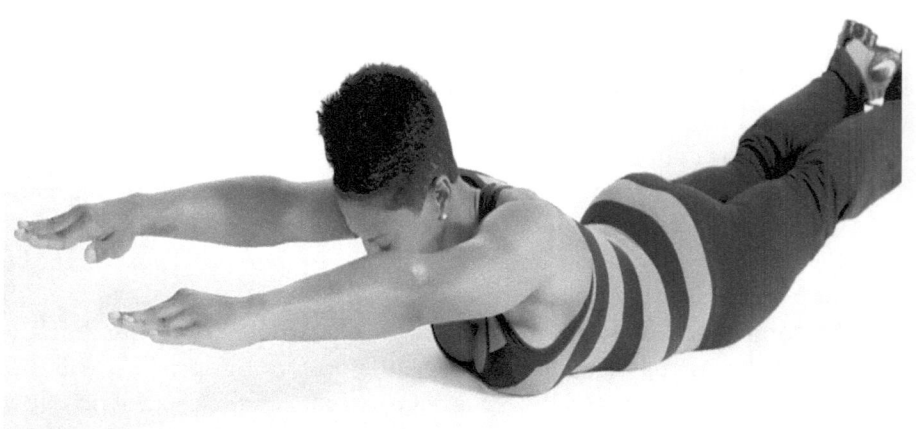

FINISH

Lowerback

Hyper extensions Manual- These can be performed 3 ways as well. The first way is on the manual hyper extension machine. Knees should be in the middle of the knee pad. Your waist should be able to bend forward and in a downward motion comfortably.

Hyper extension machine- This is another option for you. Face forward, feet on feet pedals with your back on the pad. This pad should be on the back up at about the shoulders. More support is given by this machine then the previous machine where it was all you doing the work. You will need to adjust your resistance and height of the pedals as needed. As opposed to going forward over pads, you will push the pads backward. Start from a forward seated position and push the resistance back until your body is aligned. Again, while performing controlled movements.

Superman/Superwoman- Start by laying flat on your stomach with your arms are straight forward and your legs are straight back. From this position raise both your arms and legs simultaneously for a 2-4 count depending on your speed and squeeze. Finish by lowering both your arms and legs to the floor. (OOOOH feel the burn).

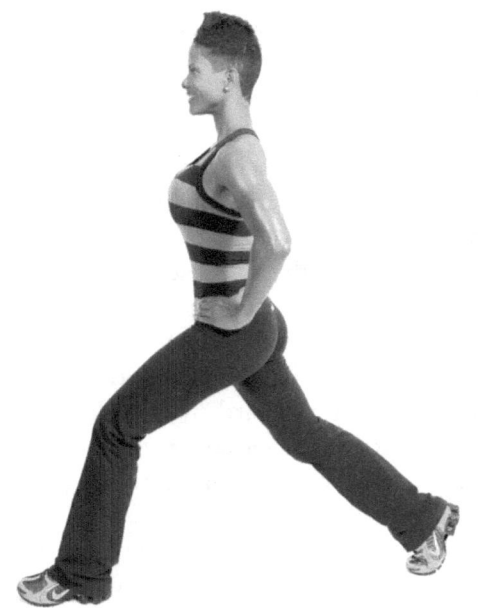

START

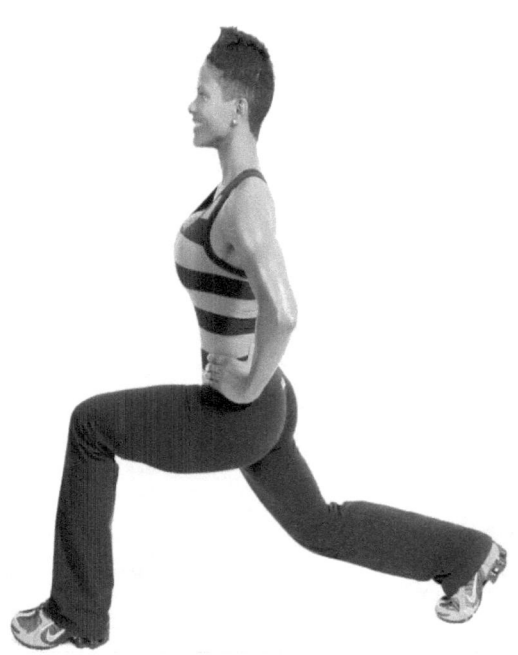

FINISH

Legs

My second favorite body part to exercise :0)
Extended walking Lunges- Great exercise to use because you are working the entire leg. Start by positioning yourself in a standing position. Your legs will be in a split position, slightly bent and extended. There should be more space between your legs than a normal lunge. The exact length depends on making sure your hind leg is stretched back comfortable enough to incorporate more space without the knee of the front leg going over the toes. One leg is forward and the other leg is backward. Next, lower yourself almost to the ground then rise back to start position. Your weight needs to be on your heel of the leg in forward position. You will push yourself up whit this heel back to starting position. Now put the leg that was in the back forward by normal walking motion then perform your lung. You will alternate each leg. Your body is your resistance, however if you feel you need more use dumbbells.

Calf Raises- These can be performed with a machine or without.

Without the machine you can go to a wall and position your hands flat on that wall. This is used for balance while on the balls of your feet at your start your body will be aligned in a straight line standing straight up. From this position rise on your toes, then back down to starting position. Seated Calf Machine- your start you are position seated on this machine with the balls of your feet and toes on the platform. Rise up on your tip toes and back down. You choose the resistance and keep these movements controlled.

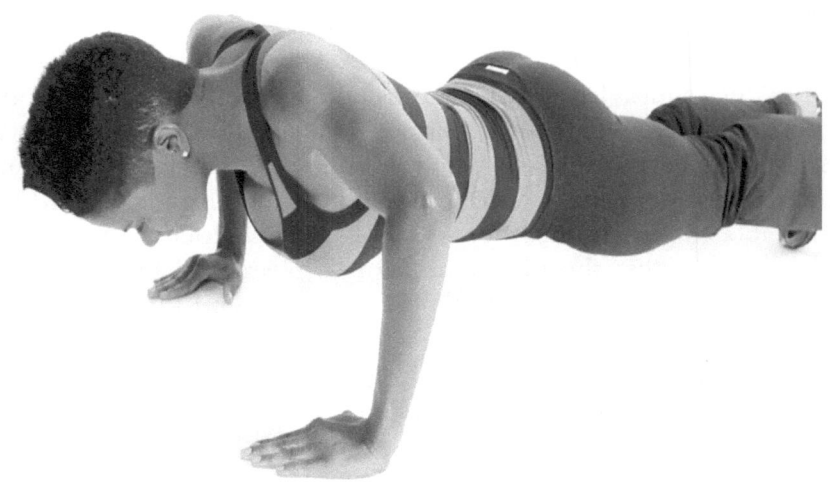

START

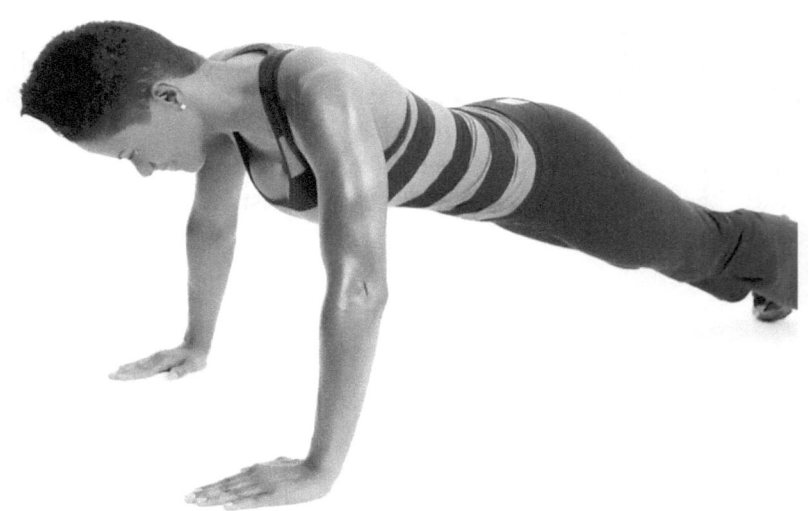

FINISH

Basic Upper Body

These can also be performed with or without machines. Well, except the pushups :0)

Pushups- This is a personal old favorite of mine because it trains a lot of the upper body in just this one exercise. 12 repetitions to start should work well. Build your way up so that you are doing 15 for the SUPERWOMEN to 20 for you SUPERMEN by the end of your 3rd week. You can do it!

Your start has you lying chest down with your palms flat on the floor a little more than shoulder width apart. Feet need to be parallel and straight. Push yourself up away from the floor while keeping your body in a straight line. This means no arching of the back. Lower your self just above the floor and repeat. You want to almost touch the floor with your chin.

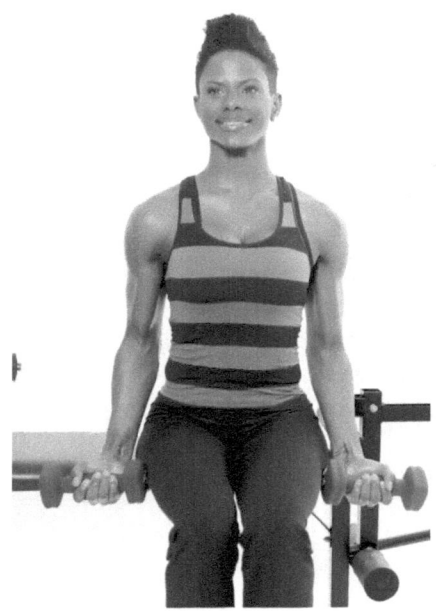

START

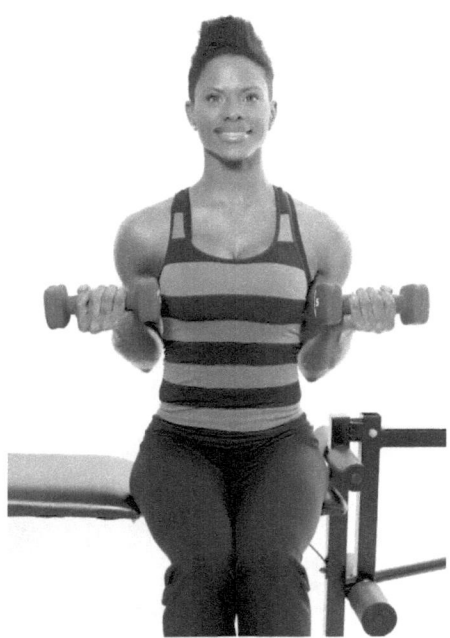

FINISH

Bicep Curl

I perform these seated. Sit at a bench on a ball or even in a chair with dumbbells. The arms are straight down at your sides for the start while your elbows are in at your sides. Elbows should not move from this fixed position. Now raise the dumbbells up to a 90 degree angle while tightening the muscle for your count. After your count lower the weight back down and stopping just before you reach straight elbows.

Bicep Curl Machine- Sit on a bicep machine with your elbows fixed on the pad. Raise the weight up towards you until you reach the 90 degree angle and release back down to almost straight elbows. This is performed like the regular bicep curl exercise.

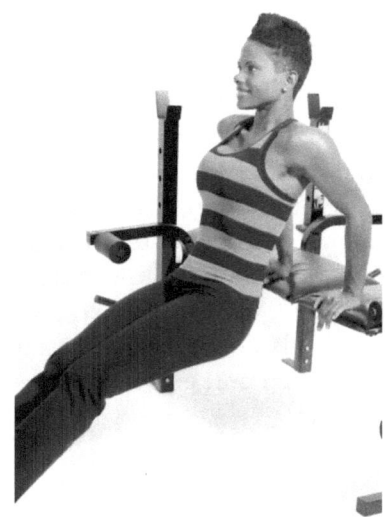

START

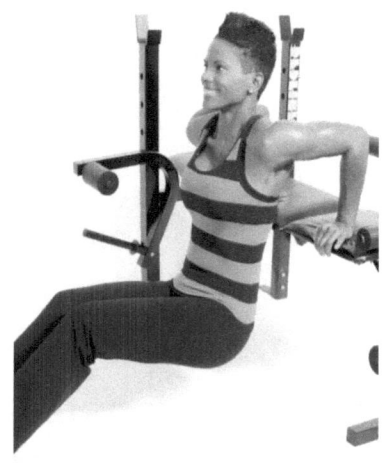

FINISH

Triceps

Training these muscles finishes the full package of that upper body.

Triceps Dip- Without a machine you will need to sit on the edge of a chair or bench tat can hold your body weight. Your hands need to be placed next to you on the chair facing forward. Lift your bottom off of the chair while lowering yourself toward the floor. Finish by raising your self up towards the chair and repeat the motion.

Triceps Dip Machine- Place yourself on this machine wit your knees on the pad facing forward and hands on the bars. Your arms will parallel each other at a 90 degree angle for the start. Now with your back straight pus yourself up until your arms or almost straight ten lower yourself back to starting position and repeat.

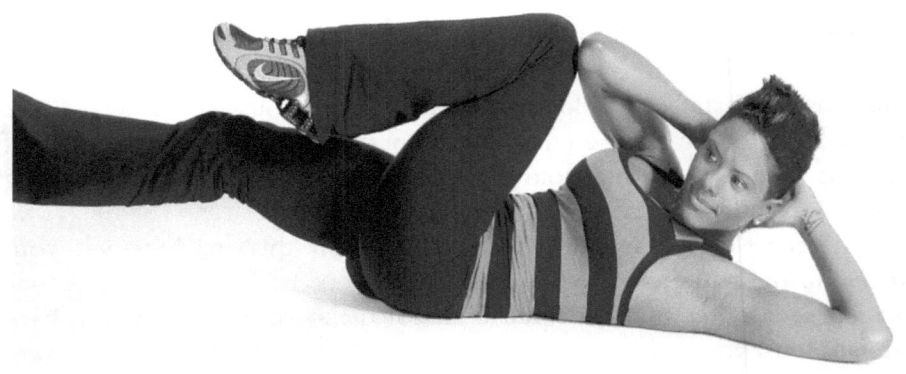

START

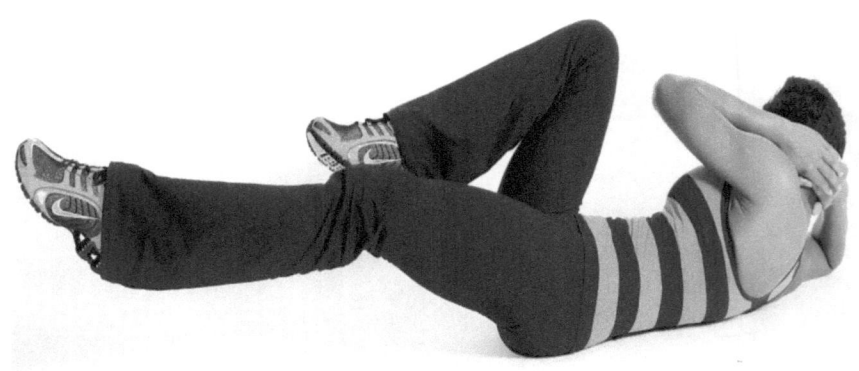

FINISH

Abs

Abs are the core of our bodies. A strong core means a better supported back, straighter posture and a centered you. While I feel it is necessary to train these muscles, I disagree with those who say its okay to train them daily because they are smaller muscles. Just like the rest of the muscles you train, the ab muscles also need rest. So my suggestion is to train the abs 2-3 times a week max. The one day on, 2 days off for those training 3 times a week.

With rest come stronger and better developed ab muscles. Everyone has ABS… EVERYONE! It is just a matter of ridding the fat hiding those beautiful muscles. Here are 2 basic exercises for the abs…

Crunches- Lay Flat on your back with your hands lightly behind your head, knees bent and feet flat on the floor. Raise your upper back off of the floor. You will raise the shoulder blades about 1 or 2 inches off the ground. While doing this squeeze and contract the ab muscles while keeping the lower back flat on the floor. Squeeze and hold at the top of the movement for a couple of seconds then lower your upper back fat to the ground.

Bicycle- Lay flat on your back with your knees bent and rose at about a 45 degree angle. Bring you right elbow towards your left knee. Then switch and bring your left elbow towards your right knee. Your legs will be moving as if you are pedaling a bike.

CARDIO

I gave you exercises for cardio in the first booklet. However, please note that cardio in conjunction with resistance is equally important to reaching you physique and or weight goals. There are many ways to prevent plateauing during your cardio sessions such as changing the actual amount of time you perform cardio to actually changing the equipment you perform on. These are positive and stimulating changes for the body.

For instance, you choose to change the amount of time you perform your exercise. Do so by increasing the length of time by 15 minutes extra. If you choose to change the resistance on the cardio machine you are using, you will increase your resistance by going 2 notches up on resistance. You will do this for 2 minutes then lower back to your starting resistance for 1 minute. This interval will be done for the total duration of your exercise.

Another great way to add change is by changing the actual cardio you perform every 2-3 weeks. If you choose to run for 20 mins, stop for a couple weeks. Instead hit the elliptical, Stairmaster or bike for 20-30 minutes.

SMILE SUPERHUMANS :0) the results are phenomenal. After 2- 3 weeks change! change! change! The only constant should be RESULTS.

MY # 1 TIP

The most important tip I can give are actual 2 tips because they are equally important in reaching your weight management goals.

BREATHE AND REST

Too many people do not breathe while performing exercises. Stop holding your breath. The muscles need the oxygen. The deeper the breath the better :0)

Rest is a must. There are also those group of people who are extreme, too extreme when it comes to how often they workout. Yes, even me at times. So for those who train 6-7 days a week you are not fallowing your body to fully rest and heal for the workouts. This leads to fatigue during your next workouts and even lowering the immune system. What happens next is the big no no. PLATEAU. None of us desire that so take 2 days extra off once a month if not more. I actually take 5-7 consecutive days off a month to let my body rest.

LOL DEFINED IN ACTION

We have come to the end of Logistics of Leanness DEFINED. However on a closing note, SUPERWOMEN and SUPERMEN, you can only succeed in reaching your goal after reading this. You are left this booklet having more POWER/KNOWLEDGE than you did before. I expect no less than what you should expect from yourself. 100% effort. After all it is your body and you deserve to have this body at its best. They say super woman and man are powerless if placed by KRYPTONITE. Fear, HEROS, is your kryptonite. Do not doubt yourself. Conquer your fears of failure and you make failure powerless. This leaves you with only the POWER to SUCCEED.

LIGHTNLOVE,

Leigh Hickombottom

www.ingramcontent.com/pod-product-compliance
Lightning Source LLC
Chambersburg PA
CBHW061226280526
45784CB00006B/2654